RETURN OF T

NOSE MASKS

By Rick Meyerowitz

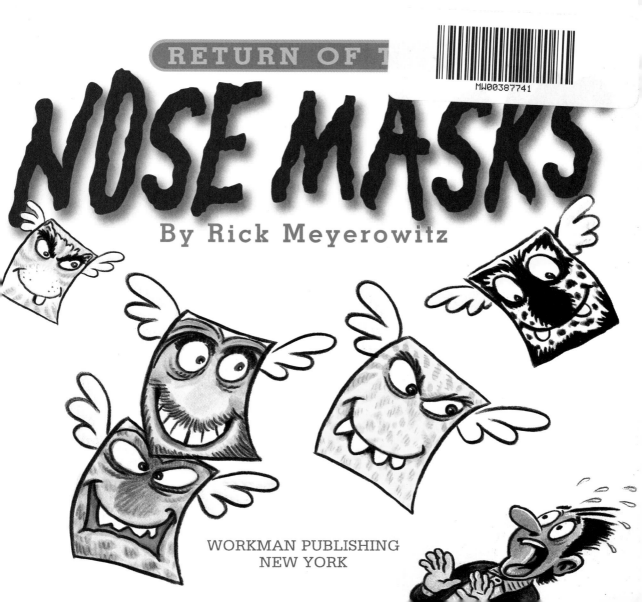

WORKMAN PUBLISHING
NEW YORK

A Message from the Author

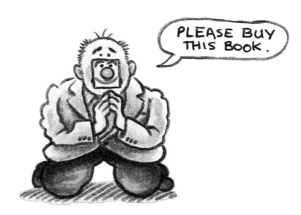

Library of Congress Cataloging-in-Publication Data

Meyerowitz, Rick

The Return of the Nose Masks

ISBN 0-7611-1244-8

1. Masks to be worn on the nose

2. Humor

Workman books are available at special discounts when purchased in bulk for premiums and sales promotions as well as for fund-raising or educational use. Special editions or book excerpts can be created to specification. For details, contact the Special Sales Director at the address below.

Workman Publishing
708 Broadway
New York, NY 10003-9555

Manufactured in the United States of America

First printing September 1998

10 9 8 7 6 5 4 3 2 1

Introduction

The first nose mask was invented shortly after the appearance of the first nose. Early men and women believed the nose to be the center of the soul. They worshiped or feared noses (usually depending on who the nose was attached to). Nose masks quickly became symbols of social status. The upper classes proudly celebrated their noses with flamboyant masks often made of ostrich feathers and garlic. Those lower on the social ladder made do with crude masks of bark, sap, and crabgrass.

Sadly, these early masks have not survived. We have only their vestigial shadows on cave walls to allow us a peek at this first burst of the human creative spirit.

In time, the blossoming of that spirit would produce such creations as *General T'ang's Nose Mask* (made of chicken feet); *Le Masque Mink de la Nez,* which Napoleon kept in his coat and pulled out on special occasions; the fabulous *Clockwork Nose Mask* that Fabergé created for Czar Nicholas, which not only kept perfect time, but fed him caviar from a golden spoon every hour; and Babe Ruth's amazing *Louisville Sneezer,* crafted out of 60 cocktail franks (now in a refrigerator at the Baseball Hall of Fame).

Wearing a nose mask tells the world that you know who you are. Wearing one is not a denial of your nose, it is an affirmation of yourself.

A final note: Nose masks are for wearing. *You are supposed to tear up this book.* If you insist on saving it intact for your collection, buy two!

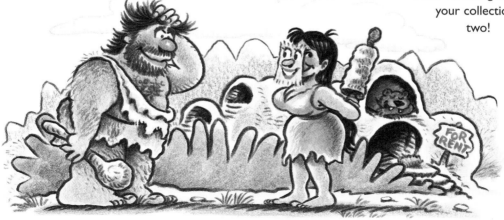

**Early gal wove nose masks from grass to attract early guy. The result?
Just the whole darn human race, that's all!**

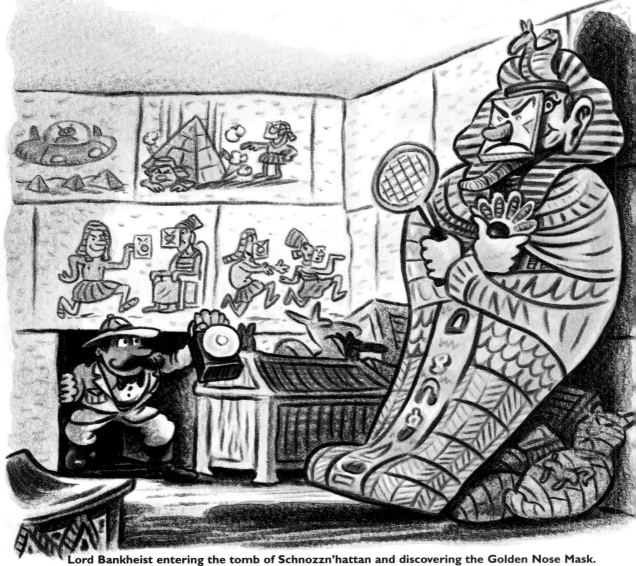

Lord Bankheist entering the tomb of Schnozzn'hattan and discovering the Golden Nose Mask. (Now in the collection of Ransack House, Oxford.)

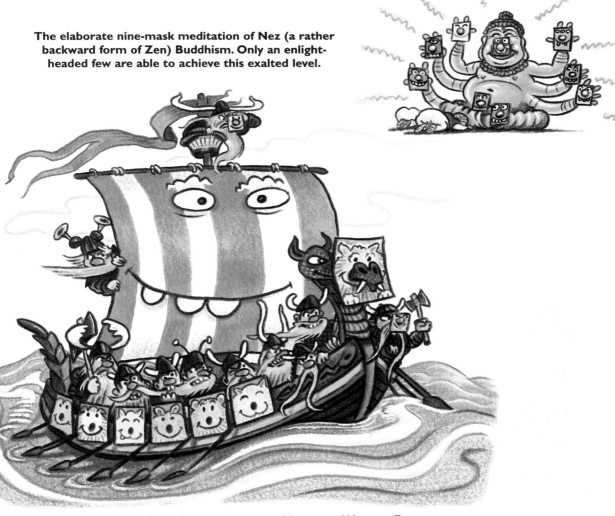

The elaborate nine-mask meditation of Nez (a rather backward form of Zen) Buddhism. Only an enlight-headed few are able to achieve this exalted level.

For centuries, fierce Nosemen wreaked havoc on Western Europe. They hid their real intentions behind nose masks. The Celts described them this way: "happy faces—sharp axes."

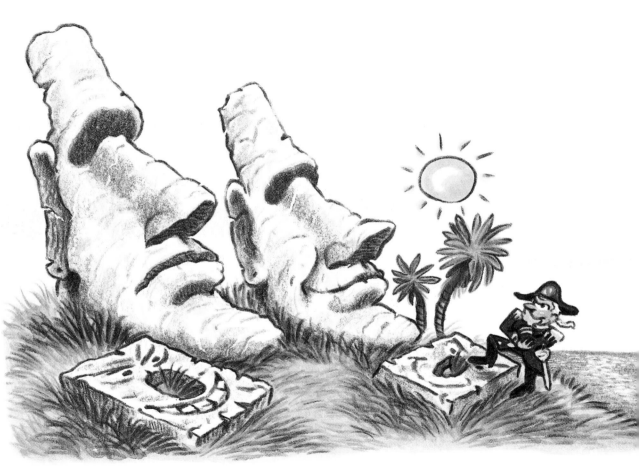

Captain Cook discovered them, but who made them, and why? Back in England, when he claimed they were nose masks, he was laughed out of Parliament, and the king called him "Captain Kook."

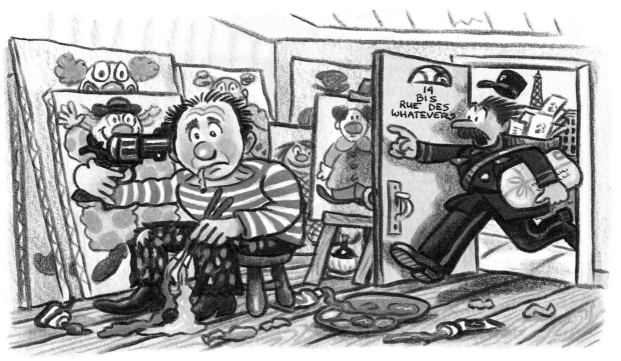

By 1905, Picasso felt he had come to a creative impasse. He was about to shoot himself when M. Choucroute, the postman, arrived with a package of rare African nose masks. Picasso revived, painted *Les Demoiselles d'Avignon,* and was never at a loss for ideas again!

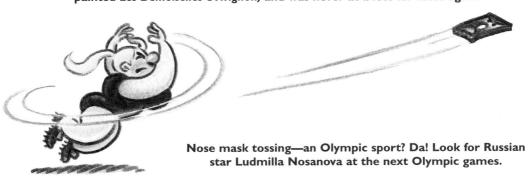

Nose mask tossing—an Olympic sport? Da! Look for Russian star Ludmilla Nosanova at the next Olympic games.

Instructions

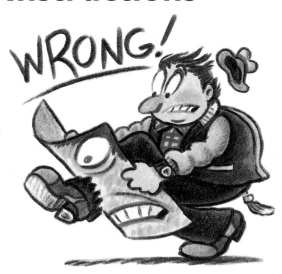

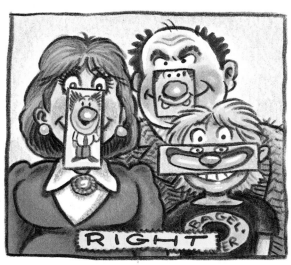

How to tear and wear a nose mask.

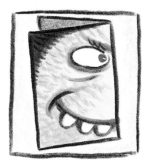

1. Gently fold mask down center.

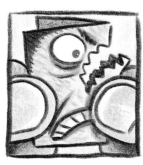

2. Tear a hole (not too wide).

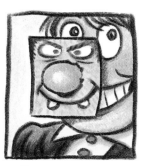

3. Place securely on nose.

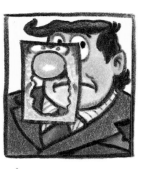

4. Start with a small hole. You can always make it larger.

Amphora Boogie

Nefretootsie

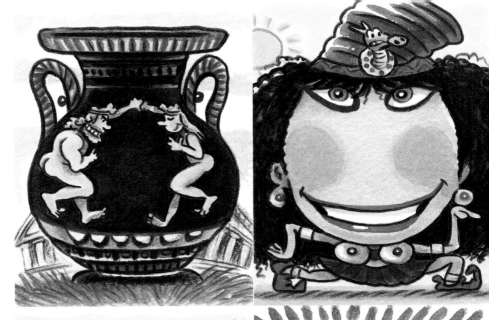

**Schnozzn'hattan
(Tootnose III)**

Doctor Zeus

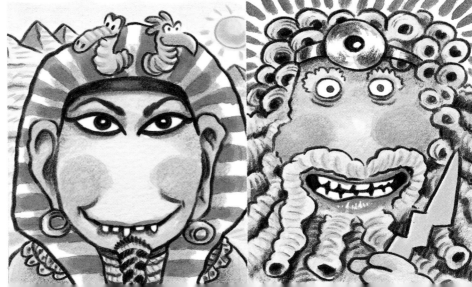

Nefretootsie

Amphora Boogie

Doctor Zeus

**Schnozzn'hattan
(Tootnose III)**

Big Bad Buddha

Kissin' Courtesan

Mahat Matowel

Sy O'Nara

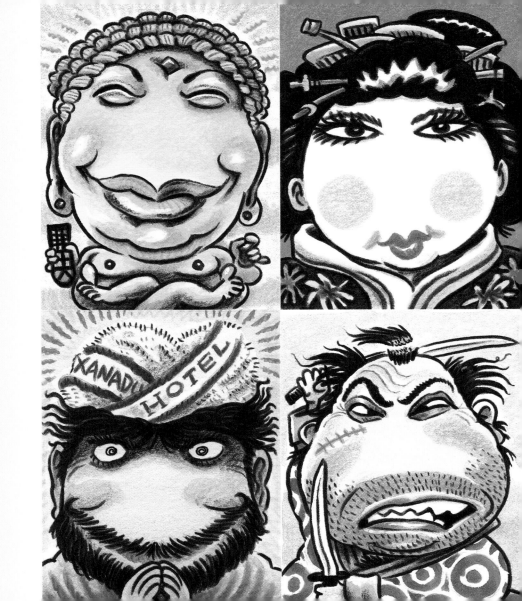

Kissin' Courtesan

Big Bad Buddha

Sy O'Nara

Mahat Matowel

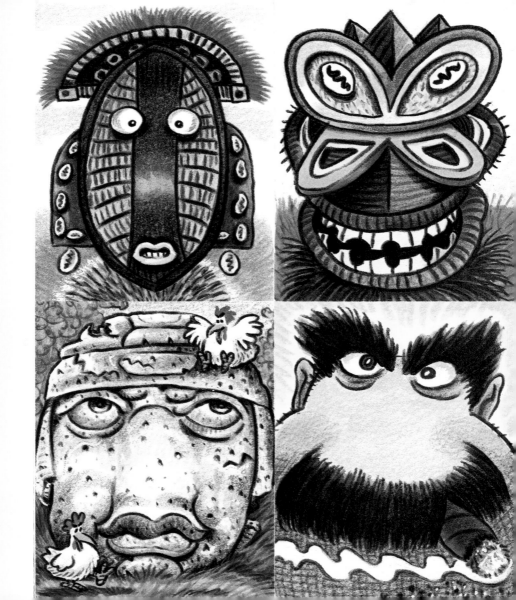

Zanzi Barbara

Olduvai George

Olmec Head
with Chickens

The Man from
Grouchistan

Olduvai George

Zanzi Barbara

The Man from
Grouchistan

Olmec Head with Chickens

Zippo

Harpo

Chicko

Gummo

Harpo

Zippo

Gummo

Chicko

M. Le Pipe

Girlnica

La Demoiselle de Nez

Bull Desiring to Be
a Nose Mask

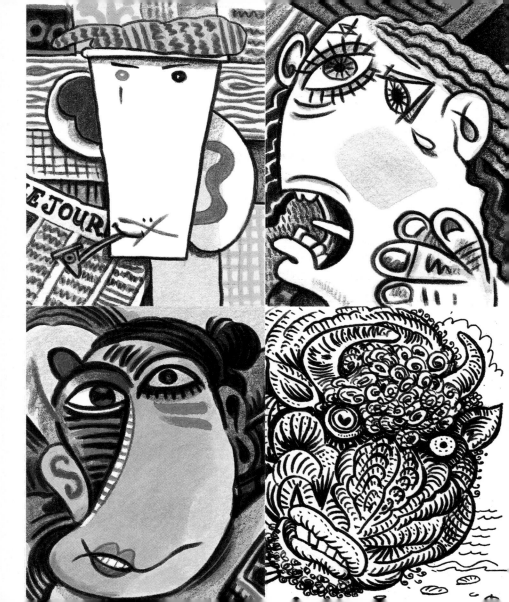

Girlnica

M. Le Pipe

Bull Desiring to Be
a Nose Mask

La Demoiselle de Nez

Spotzie

Sniffy

Pumpsie

Orange Julius

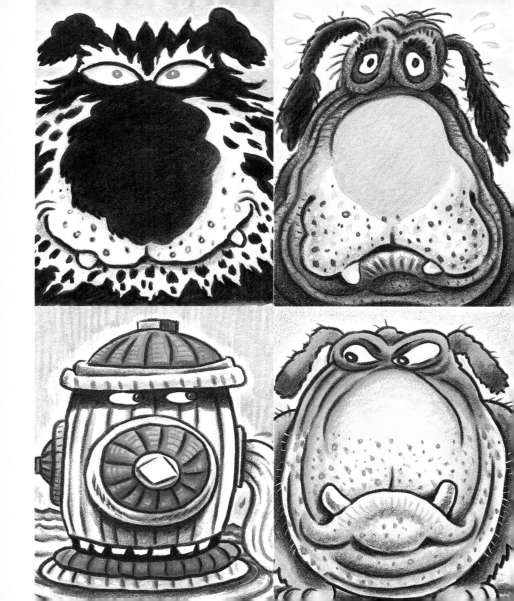

Sniffy

Spotzie

Orange Julius

Pumpsie

Vincent and…

Velma of Verona

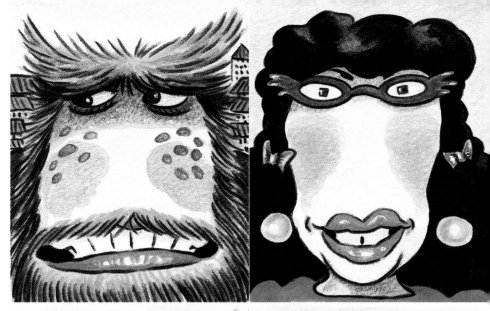

Lawrence and…

Lenore of Arabia

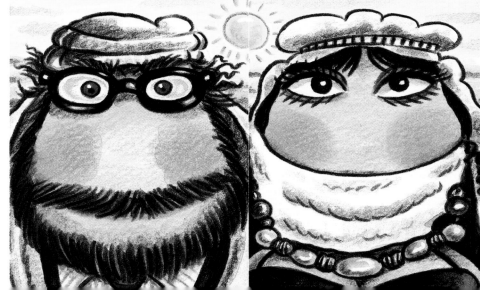

Velma and…   Vincent of Verona

Lenore and…   Lawrence of Arabia

Ol' Granny Smith

Pomme de Terrible

Mac

Johnny Appleface

Pomme de Terrible

Ol' Granny Smith

Johnny Appleface

Mac

Gretta Crabbo

Ethyl Mermaid

J. Edgar Guppy

The Octoputtz

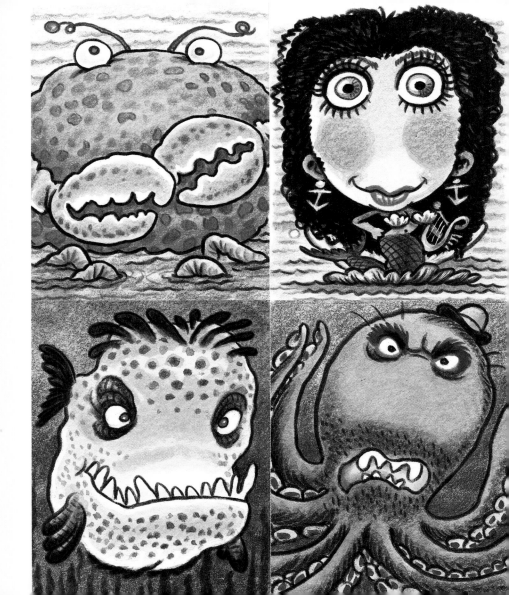

Ethyl Mermaid

Gretta Crabbo

The Octoputtz

J. Edgar Guppy

Gina

Olaf

Mick

Pierre (Le Frog Bleu)

Olaf

Gina

Pierre (Le Frog Bleu)

Mick

Orson Lard

Lauren Bacon

Charlie Choplin

Brad Pork

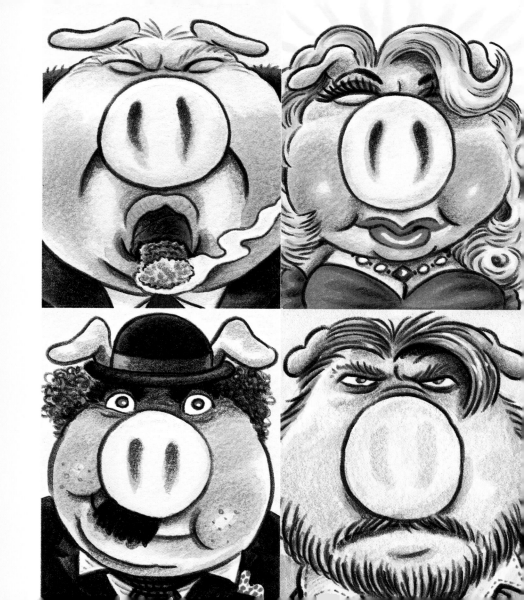

Lauren Bacon

Orson Lard

Brad Pork

Charlie Choplin

MacChew

McPunt

McSneaker Contract

MacPuck

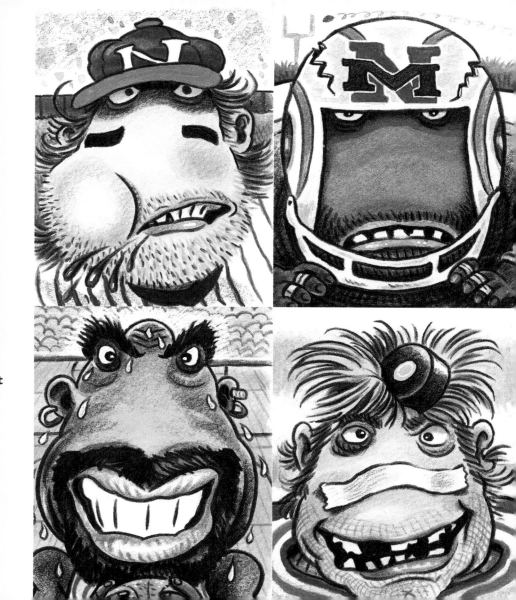

McPunt

MacChew

MacPuck

McSneaker Contract

Cocktail Cat

Fat Cat

Cool Cat

Morris Katz

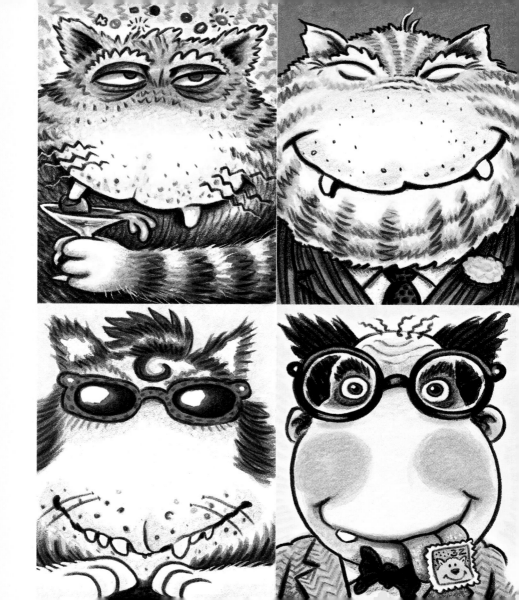

Fat Cat

Cocktail Cat

Morris Katz

Cool Cat

Rudy Croody

Teasin' Tessie

Daddy's Girl

Mummy's Boy

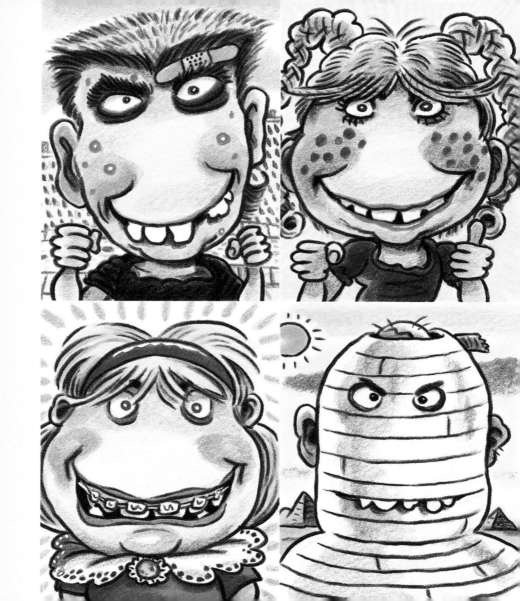

Teasin' Tessie

Rudy Croody

Mummy's Boy

Daddy's Girl

The Velvet Frog

Bee-Bopper

American Flyer

Bugged Out!

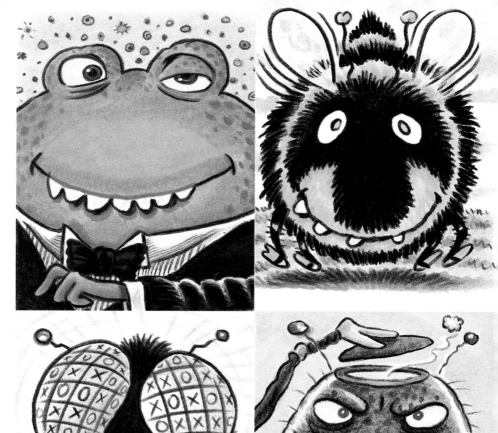
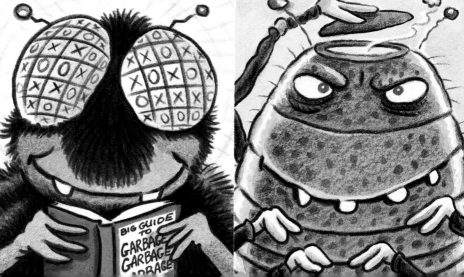

Bee-Bopper

The Velvet Frog

Bugged Out!

American Flyer

Pizza Face

Pepper Puss

Tough Cookie

3-Minute Menace

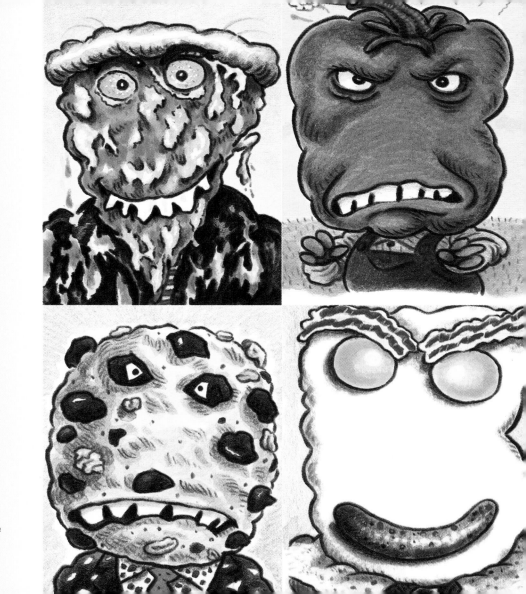

Pepper Puss

Pizza Face

3-Minute Menace

Tough Cookie

Crying Baby

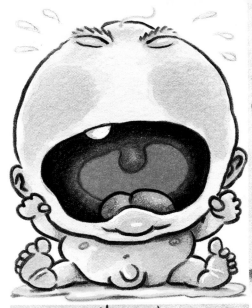

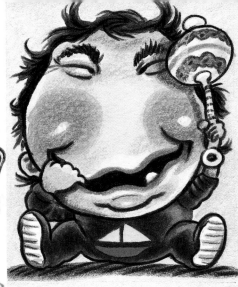

Laughing Baby

Pretty Baby

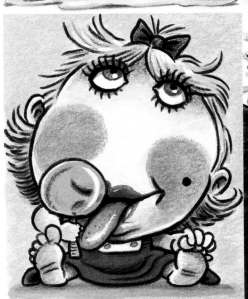

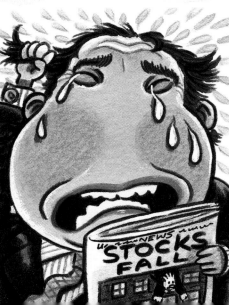

Big Baby

Laughing Baby   **Crying Baby**

Big Baby   **Pretty Baby**

Cyclutz

Dubble Trubble

Triclops

Ol' Four Eyes

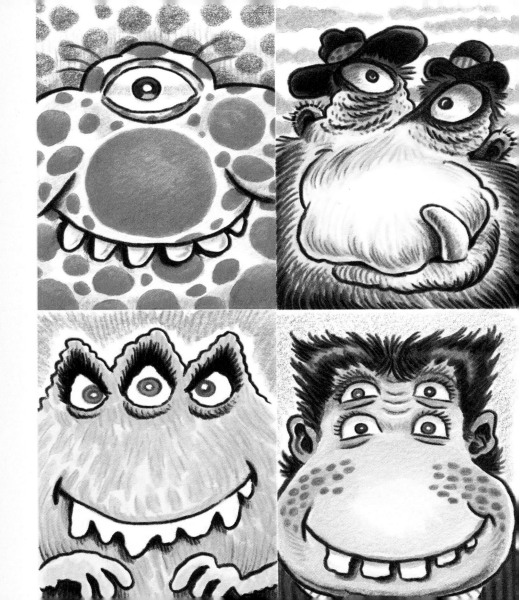

Dubble Trubble

Cyclutz

Ol' Four Eyes

Triclops

Snorky

Ms. Schwimmer

Somethin' Fishy

Felix

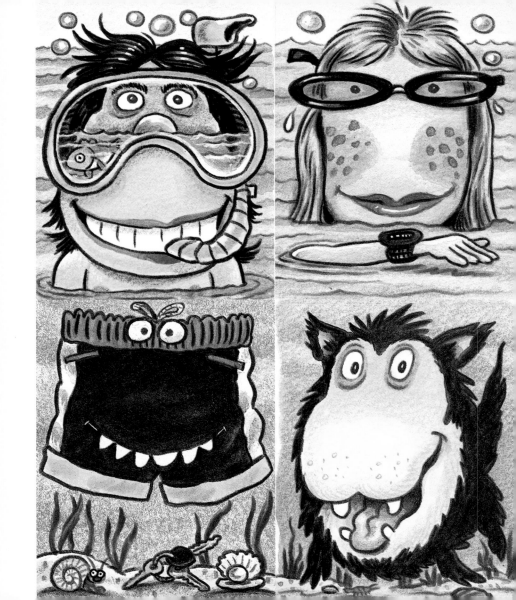

Ms. Schwimmer

Snorky

Felix

Somethin' Fishy

Ph.D.

M.D.

C.P.A.

Esq.

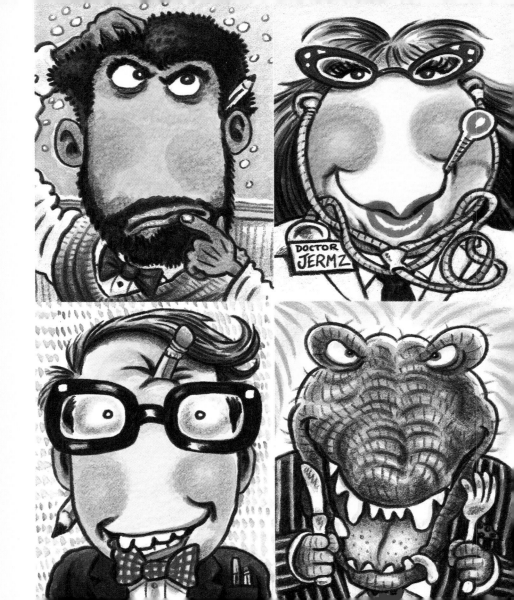

M.D.

Ph.D.

Esq.

C.P.A.

Biff Stroganoff

Doris Yeltsin

Indiana Bones

Tiffannee

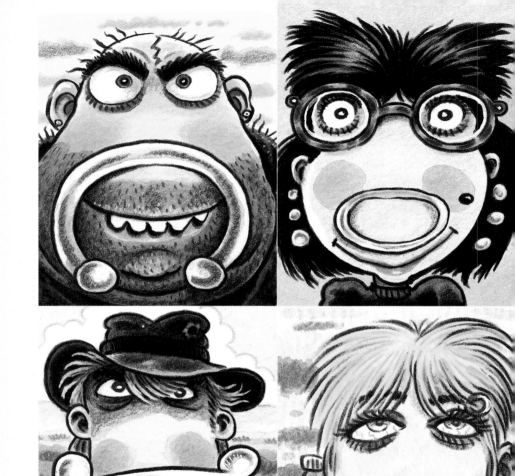

Doris Yeltsin

Biff Stroganoff

Tiffannee

Indiana Bones

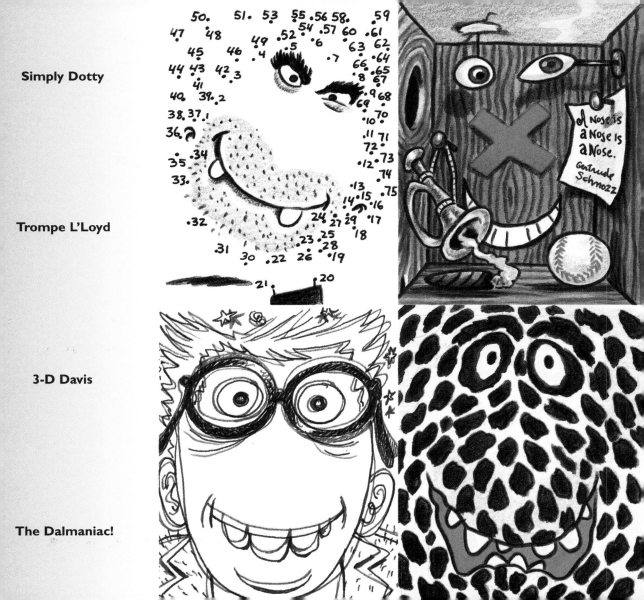

Simply Dotty

Trompe L'Loyd

3-D Davis

The Dalmaniac!

Trompe L'Loyd

Simply Dotty

The Dalmaniac!

3-D Davis

La Targeta

La Escreama

El Brewski

El Igloo

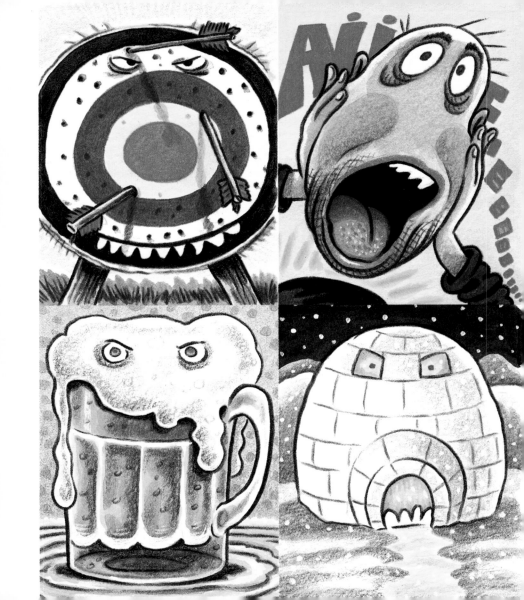

La Escreama

La Targeta

El Igloo

El Brewski

Wolfgang Pucker

www.nose.con

The Tie

Uncle!

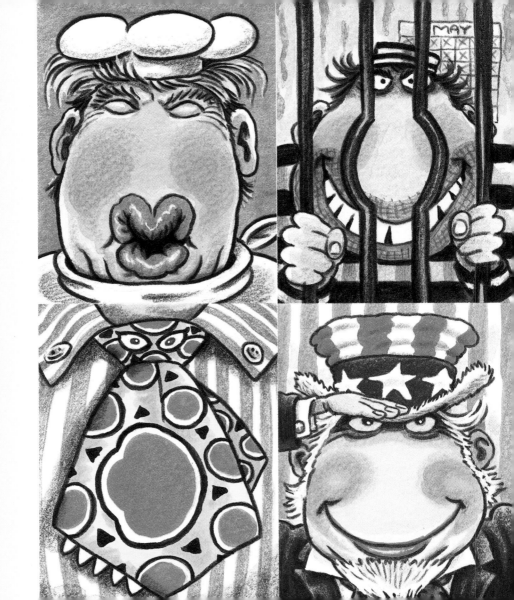

www.nose.con

Wolfgang Pucker

Uncle!

The Tie

Wanda Witchell

Gobbles

Hollow Harry

Hallow Inky

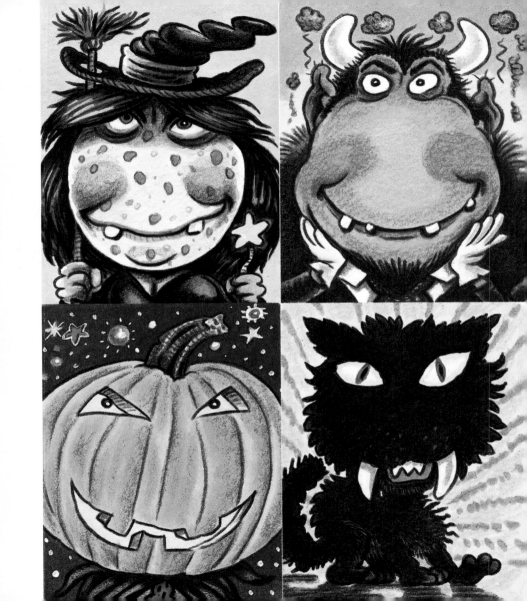

Gobbles

Wanda Witchell

Hallow Inky

Hollow Harry

Peaches

Cute 'n' Fuzzy

Blitzen,
James Blitzen

The Angel of Death!

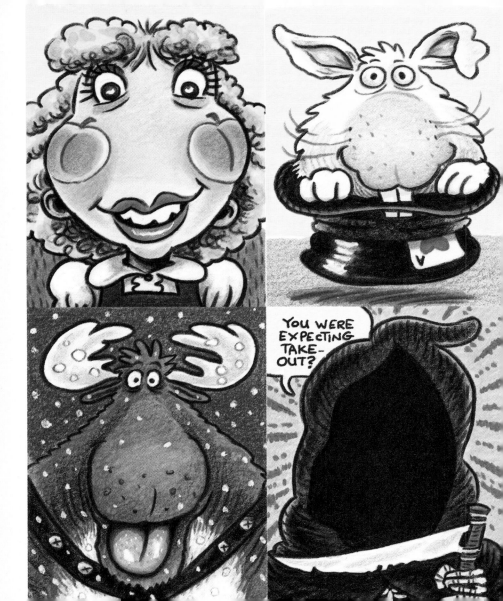

Cute 'n' Fuzzy

Peaches

The Angel of Death!

Blitzen,
James Blitzen

Arrggghh!
by Van Gogh

Portrait of My Nose
by Rembrandt

Le Conosedrum
by Magritte

Day of the Schnozzle
by Dali

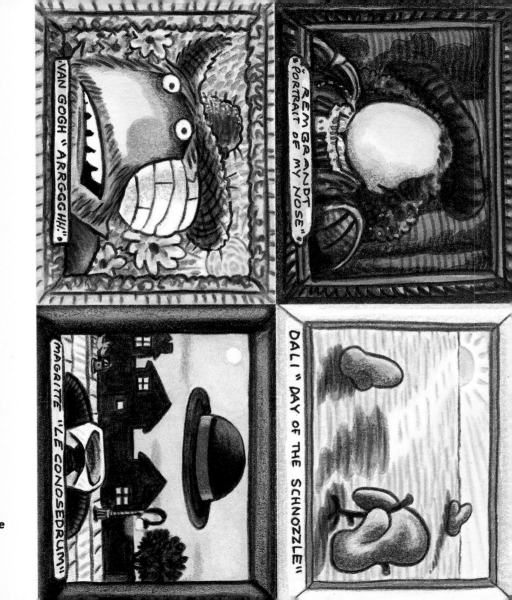

Portrait of My Nose
by Rembrandt

Arrggghh!
by Van Gogh

Day of the Schnozzle
by Dali

Le Conosedrum
by Magritte

"Hey, you!"

"Hello, Earthling."

"Well, hi there."

"Hello! I'm…"

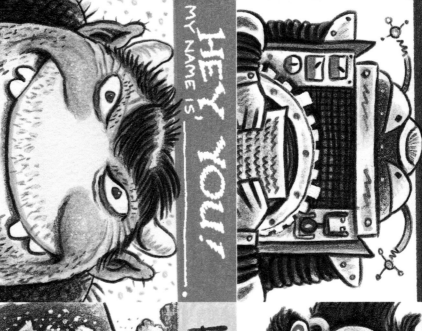

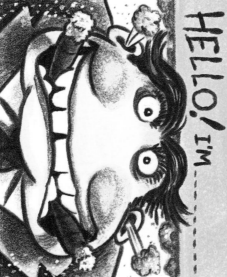

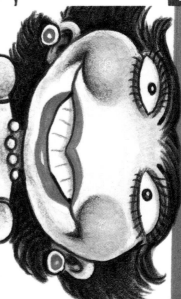

"Hello, Earthling."

"Hey, you!"

"Well, hi there."

"Hello! I'm…"

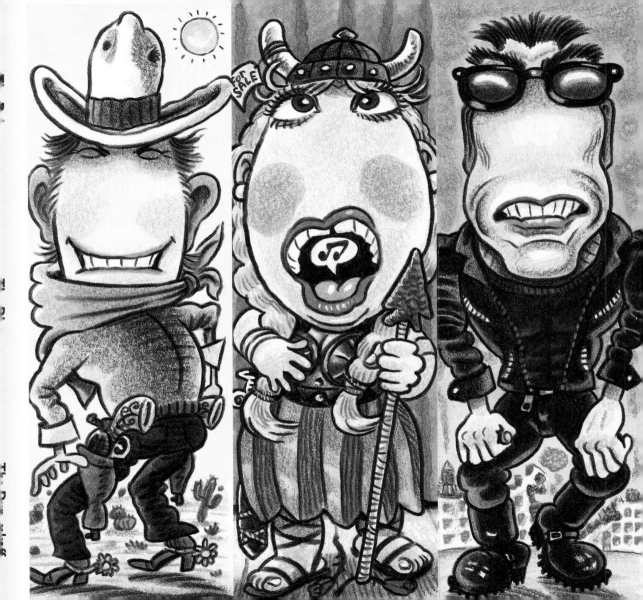

The Dummkoff   **The Diva**   **The Duke**

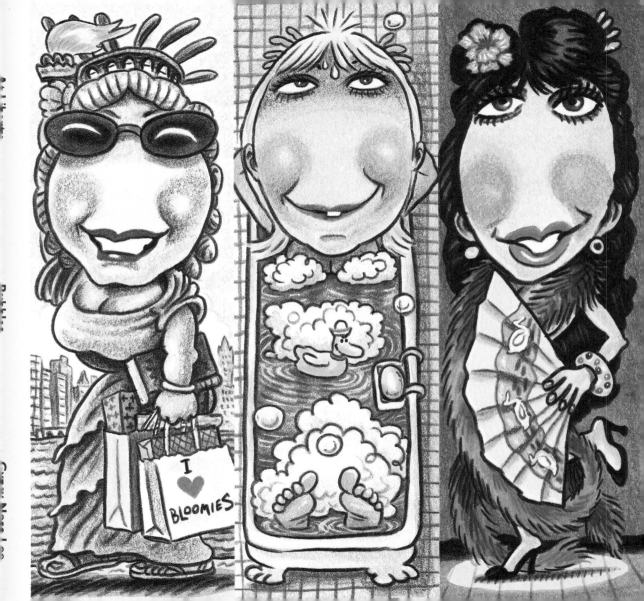

Gypsy Nose Lee   **Bubbles**   **At Liberty**

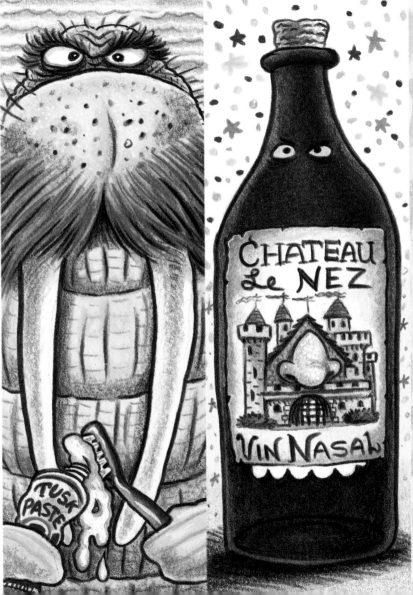

Magnum Faure

Bananarama

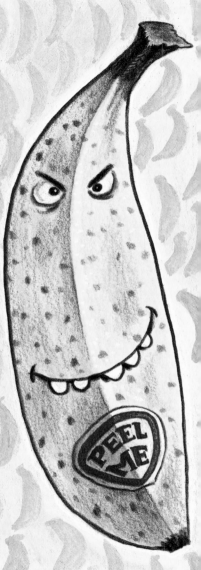

Bananarama   Magnum Farce   Big Wally

Il Fazzo

La Prima Donna

Da Pelvis

Da Pelvis   La Prima Donna   Il Fazzo

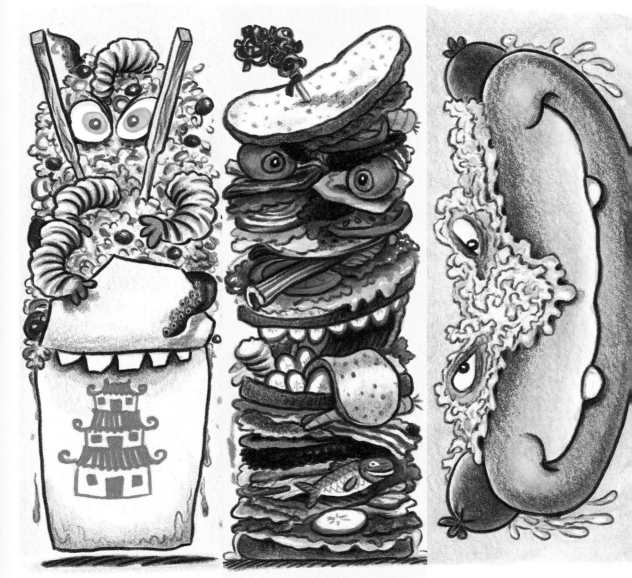

The Creature in the Rye

Dogzilla!

Dogzilla!   The Creature in the Rye   Tommy Take-Out

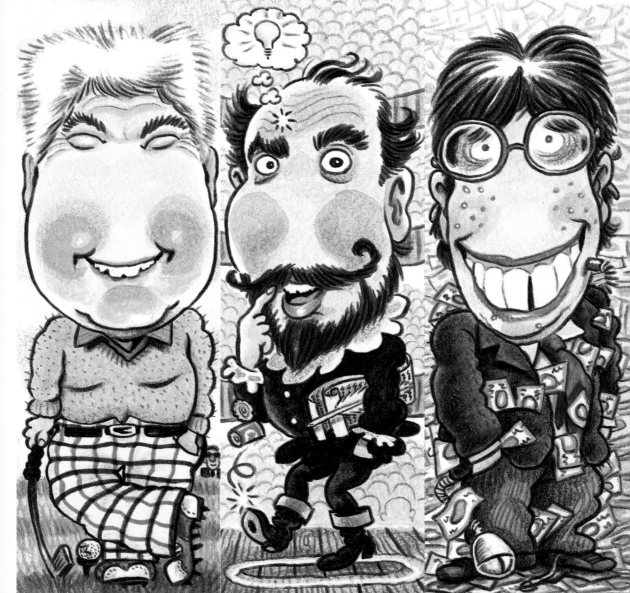

Bill Yuns   **Classic Bill**   **Big Willy**

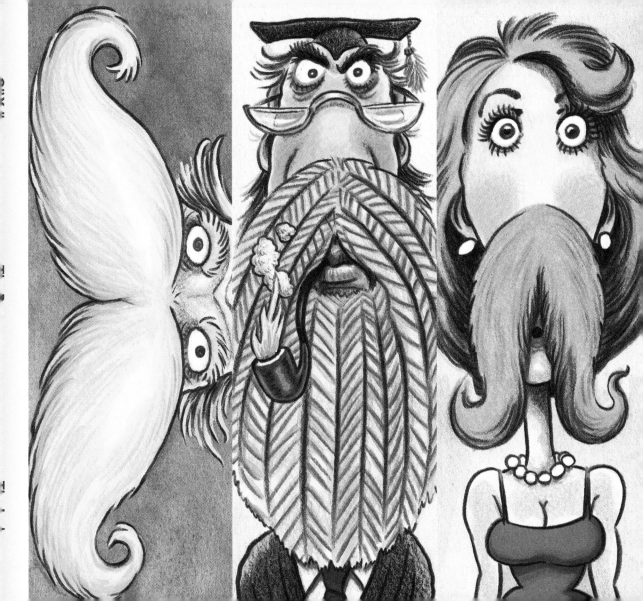

The Lady   The Perfessor   Ol' Yeller

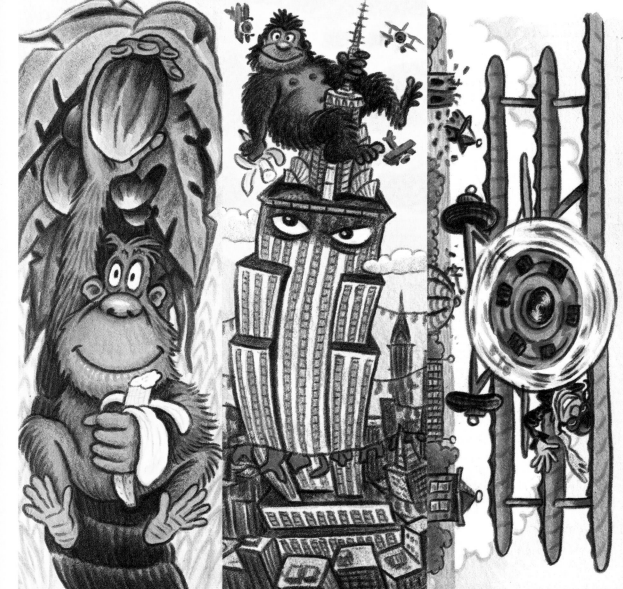

Plane Insane   Banana State Building   Monkey Biz

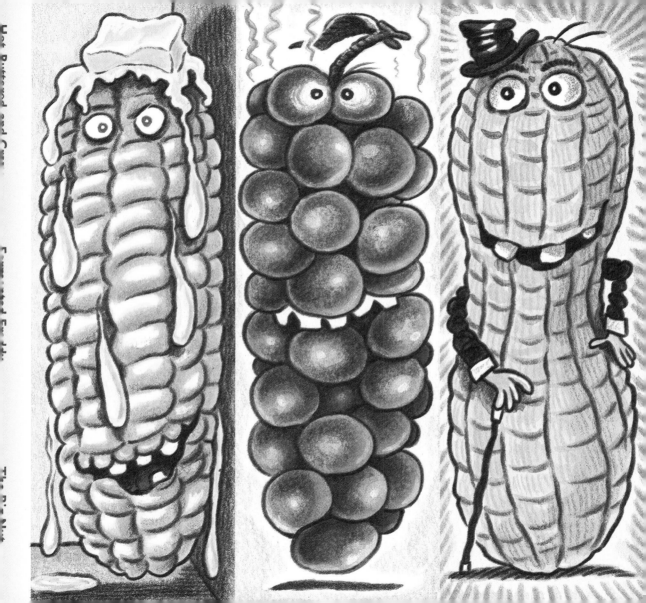

The Big Nut   Fermented Freddy   Hot, Buttered, and Crazy

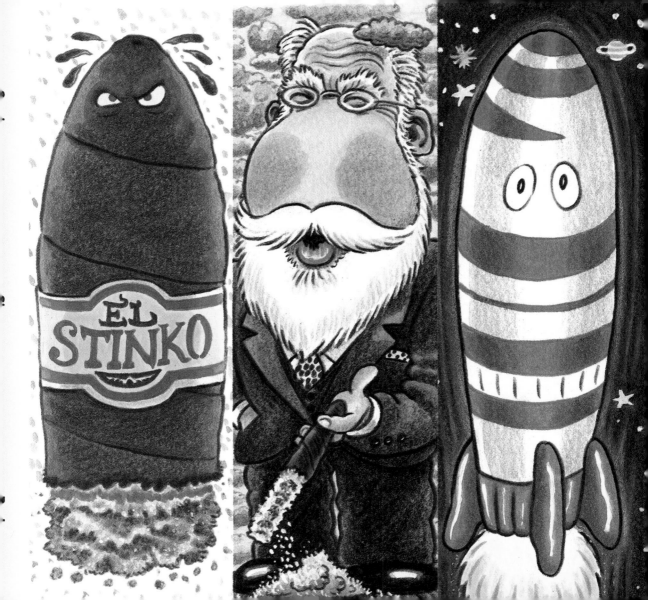

Rocky   Siggy   Stogie

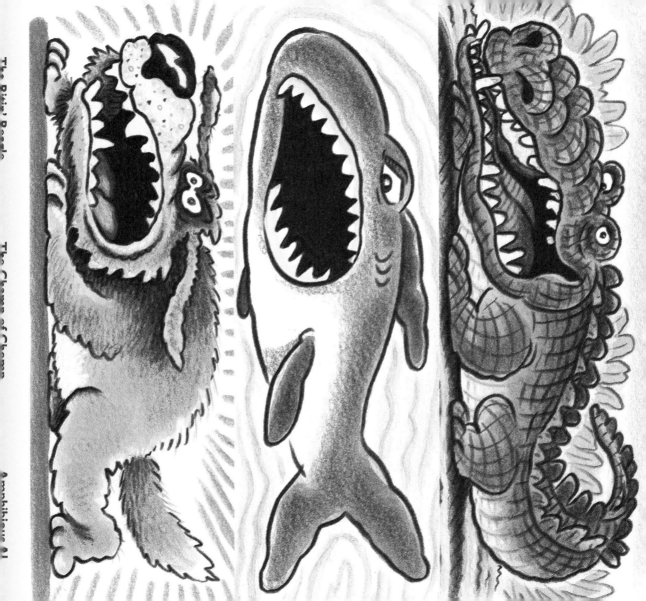

Amphibious Al   The Champ of Chomp   The Bitin' Beagle

AC/DC

Card Trip

Double Denny

Double Denny   **Card Trip**   **AC/DC**

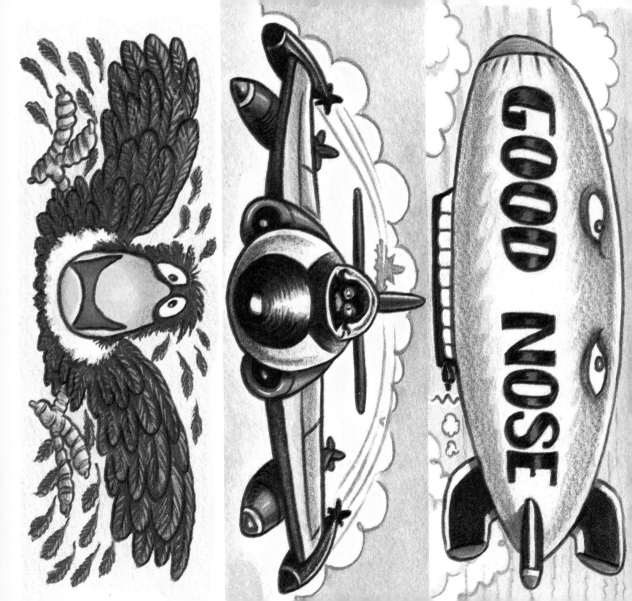

The Flying Featherneck   Nosedive!   George Blimpton

George Blimpton   Nosedive!   The Flying Featherneck

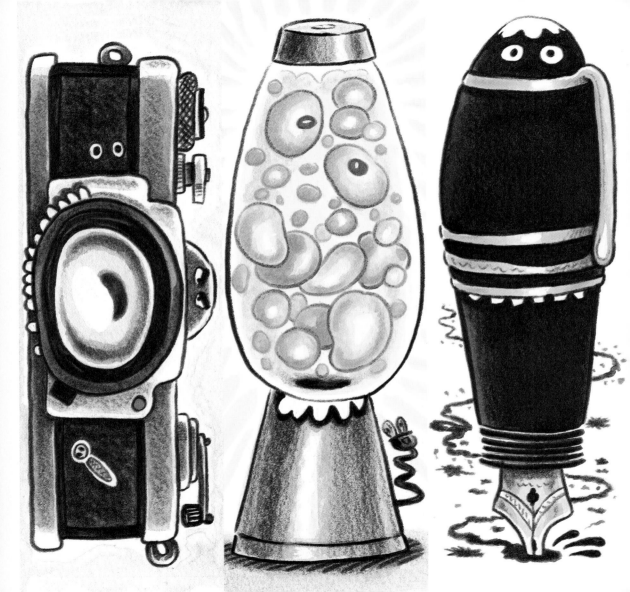

Der Scribbler   Lava Louie   F. Stop Fitzgerald

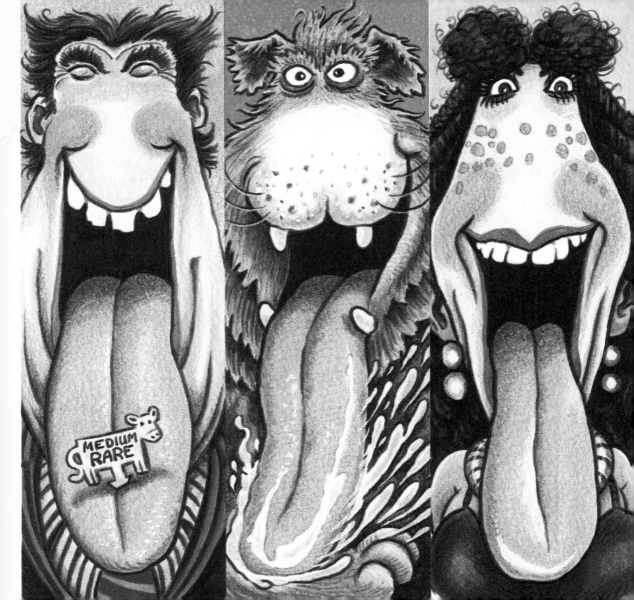

Yolanda Yeccch   Big Pink   Irving Iccch